Air Fryer Cookbook for Your Lunch & Dinner

Don't Miss These Quick and Easy Recipes to Make Incredible Air Fryer Appetizers

Kira Hamm

TABLE OF CONTENT

this book has been derived from various sources. Please consult a licensed professional before attempting any techniques outlined in this book.

By reading this document, the reader agrees that under no circumstances is the author responsible for any losses, direct or indirect, which are incurred as a result of the use of information contained within this document, including, but not limited to, — errors, omissions, or inaccuracies.

Egg Sausage Spinach Cups

Preparation Time:10 minutes

Cooking Time: 10 minutes

Servings:2

Ingredients:

1. 1/4 cup egg beaters
2. 4 tbsp sausage, cooked and crumbled
3. 4 tsp jack cheese, shredded
4. 4 tbsp spinach, chopped

Directions:

1. Spray two ramekins with cooking spray and set aside.
2. In a mixing bowl, whisk together all ingredients until well combined.
3. Pour mixture into the ramekins.
4. Place ramekins into the air fryer basket and cook at 330 F for 10 minutes.

Nutrition: Calories 306 Fat 23.4 g Carbohydrates 2.4 g Sugar 0.2 g Protein 20.9 g Cholesterol 72 mg

Breakfast Eggs Avocado

Preparation Time:10 minutes

Cooking Time: 9 minutes

Servings:2

Ingredients:

- 2 eggs
- 1 avocado, cut in half and remove the seed
- Pinch of red pepper flakes

Directions:

1. Break one egg into each avocado half. Season with red pepper flakes, pepper, and salt.
2. Place avocado halves into the air fryer basket and cook at 400 F for 5 minutes or until eggs are cooked. Check after 5 minutes.

Nutrition: Calories 268 Fat 24 g Carbohydrates 9.1 g Sugar 0.9 g Protein 7.5 g Cholesterol 164 mg

Egg Bacon Cheese Bites

Preparation Time:10 minutes

Cooking Time: 13 minutes

Servings:4

Ingredients:

- 4 eggs
- 1/4 cup cheddar cheese, shredded
- 4 bacon slices, cooked and crumbled
- 1/2 small bell pepper, diced
- 1/2 onion, diced
- 4 tsp coconut milk

Directions:

1. Spray four ramekins with cooking spray.
2. Crack 1 egg into each ramekin then adds 1 tsp coconut milk into each one.
3. Top each one off with bacon, bell pepper, onion, and cheese. Season with pepper and salt.
4. Place ramekins into the air fryer basket and cook at 300 F for 10-13 minutes.

Nutrition: Calories 216 Fat 15.9 g Carbohydrates 3.4 g Sugar 1.9 g Protein 14.8 g Cholesterol 192 mg

Egg Ham Bites

Preparation Time:10 minutes

Cooking Time: 12 minutes

Servings:8

Ingredients:

- 6 eggs
- 1/2 cup cheddar cheese, shredded
- 1 cup ham, diced
- 2 tbsp cream
- 1/4 tsp garlic powder
- 1/4 tsp onion powder

Directions:

1. In a bowl, whisk eggs with remaining ingredients.
2. Pour egg mixture into the silicone muffin molds.
3. Place molds into the air fryer basket and cook at 300 F for 12-14 minutes or until eggs are cooked.

Nutrition: Calories 106 Fat 7.2 g Carbohydrates 1.2 g Sugar 0.4 g Protein 8.8 g Cholesterol 140 mg

Egg Cheese Mustard Bake

Preparation Time: 10 minutes

Cooking Time: 25 minutes

Servings: 3

Ingredients:

- 6 eggs
- 1/4 tsp dry mustard
- 2 tbsp butter, melted
- 1/4 lb. cheddar cheese, grated
- 1/2 cup coconut milk

Directions:

1. Spray air fryer safe pan with cooking spray and set aside.
2. In a bowl, whisk eggs with milk, mustard, pepper, and salt. Stir in cheese.
3. Pour egg mixture into the pan.
4. Place pan in the air fryer basket and cook at 350 F for 25 minutes.

Nutrition: Calories 439 Fat 38.6 g Carbohydrates 3.5 g Sugar 2.3 g Protein 21.6 g Cholesterol 387 mg

Breakfast Egg Bites

Preparation Time:10 minutes

Cooking Time: 5 minutes

Servings:6

Ingredients:

- 4 eggs
- 1/4 cup cheddar cheese, shredded
- 4 tsp almond milk

Directions:

1. Spray egg bite mold with cooking spray and set aside.
2. In a bowl, whisk eggs with cheese, milk, pepper, and salt.
3. Pour egg mixture into the mold.
4. Place the mold into the air fryer basket and cook at 330 F for 5 minutes. Make sure eggs are lightly browned in color on top.
5. Serve and enjoy.

Nutrition: Calories 69 Fat 5.3 g Carbohydrates 0.5 g Sugar 0.4 g Protein 4.9 g Cholesterol 114 mg

Egg Stuffed Peppers

Preparation Time:10 minutes

Cooking Time: 13 minutes

Servings:2

Ingredients:

- 4 eggs
- 1 bell pepper, halved and remove seeds
- Pinch of red pepper flakes
- Pepper
- Salt

Directions:

1. Crack two eggs into each bell pepper half.
2. Season with red pepper flakes, pepper, and salt.
3. Place bell pepper halves into the air fryer basket and cook at 390 F for 13 minutes.
4. Serve and enjoy.

Nutrition: Calories 145 Fat 8.9 g Carbohydrates 5.3 g Sugar 3.7 g Protein 11.7 g Cholesterol 327 mg

Eggs in Bread Cups

Preparation Time: 10 m

Cooking Time: 23 m

Servings: 4

Ingredients:

- 4 bacon slices
- 2 bread slices, crust removed
- 4 eggs
- Salt and freshly ground black pepper, to taste

Directions:

1. Grease 4 cups of the muffin pan and put aside.
2. Heat a little frypan over medium-high heat and cook the bacon slices for about 2-3 minutes.
3. With a slotted spoon, transfer the bacon slice onto a paper towel-lined plate to chill.
4. Break each bread slice in half.
5. Arrange one bread slice half in each of the muffin cups and press slightly.
6. Now, arrange one bacon slice over each bread slice in a circular shape.

7. Crack one egg into each muffin cup and sprinkle with salt and black pepper.
8. Turn the "Temperature Knob" of Power XL Air Fryer Grill to line the temperature to 350 degrees F.
9. Turn the "Function Knob" to settle on "Bake."
10. Turn the "Timer Knob" to line the Time for 20 minutes.
11. After preheating, arrange the muffin pan over the roasting rack.
12. Insert the roasting rack at position 3 of the Air Fryer Grill.
13. When the cooking Time is over, remove the muffin pan and place it onto a wire rack for about 5 minutes before serving.

Nutrition: Calories: 235 Kcal, Fat: 16.7g, Carb: 3.4g, Protein 16g

Spinach Baked Eggs

Preparation Time:10 minutes

Cooking Time: 8 minutes

Servings:2

Ingredients:

- 2 eggs
- 1/4 tsp parsley, chopped
- 1/4 tsp thyme
- 1/4 tsp rosemary
- 1/4 onion, diced
- 1/4 cup spinach, chopped
- Pepper
- Salt

Directions:

1. Preheat the cosori air fryer to 350 F.
2. Spray two ramekins with cooking spray and set aside.
3. In a bowl, whisk eggs with remaining ingredients.
4. Pour egg mixture into the ramekins.
5. Place ramekins into the air fryer basket and cook for 5-8 minutes.
6. Serve and enjoy.

Nutrition: Calories 70 Fat 4.4 g Carbohydrates 2 g Sugar 0.9 g Protein 5.8 g Cholesterol 164 mg

Easy Breakfast Frittata

Preparation Time:10 minutes

Cooking Time: 15 minutes

Servings:2

Ingredients:

- 1 cup egg whites
- 1/4 cup mushrooms, sliced
- 1/4 cup tomato, sliced
- 2 tbsp coconut milk
- 2 tbsp chives, chopped

Directions:

1. Spray air fryer safe pan with cooking spray and set aside.
2. Preheat the cosori air fryer to 320 F.
3. In a bowl, whisk eggs with pepper and salt. Add remaining ingredients and mix well.
4. Pour egg mixture to the.
5. Place pan in the air fryer basket and cook for 15 minutes.

Nutrition: Calories 105 Fat 3.9 g Carbohydrates 3.1 g Sugar 2.2 g Protein 14.2 g Cholesterol 0 mg

Green Chilis Egg Bite

Preparation Time:10 minutes

Cooking Time: 5 minutes

Servings:7

Ingredients:

- 4 eggs
- 1/4 cup green chilis, diced
- 1/2 cup cottage cheese, crumbled
- 1/2 cup pepper jack cheese, shredded

Directions:

1. Spray egg mold with cooking spray and set aside.
2. In a bowl, beat eggs until frothy. Add remaining Ingredients into the eggs and stir to mix.
3. Pour egg mixture into the egg mold.
4. Place egg mold into the air fryer basket and cook at 330 F for 5 minutes.

Nutrition: Calories 57 Fat 3.1 g Carbohydrates 1.4 g Sugar 0.5 g Protein 5.5 g Cholesterol 96 mg

Roasted Pepper Egg Bite

Preparation Time:10 minutes

Cooking Time: 5 minutes

Servings:7

Ingredients:

- 4 eggs
- 1/4 cup spinach, chopped
- 1/2 roasted red pepper, chopped
- 1 tbsp green onion, chopped
- 1/2 cup cottage cheese, crumbled
- 1/2 cup Monterey jack cheese, shredded

Directions:

1. Spray egg mold with cooking spray and set aside.
2. In a bowl, beat eggs until frothy. Add remaining Ingredients into the eggs and stir to mix.
3. Pour egg mixture into the egg mold.
4. Place egg mold into the air fryer basket and cook at 330 F for 5 minutes.

Nutrition: Calories 82 Fat 5.3 g Carbohydrates 1.3 g Sugar 0.5 g Protein 7.5 g Cholesterol 102 mg

Broccoli Bell Pepper Frittata

Preparation Time:10 minutes

Cooking Time: 17 minutes

Servings:2

Ingredients:

- 3 eggs
- 2 tbsp cheddar cheese, shredded
- 2 tbsp cream
- 1/2 cup bell pepper, chopped
- 1/2 cup broccoli florets, chopped
- 1/4 tsp garlic powder
- 1/4 tsp onion powder

Directions:

1. Spray air fryer pan with cooking spray. Add bell peppers and broccoli into the pan.
2. Place pan in the air fryer basket and cook at 350 F for 7 minutes.
3. In a bowl, whisk eggs with cheese, cream, garlic powder, onion powder, pepper, and salt.
4. Pour egg mixture over broccoli and bell pepper and cook for 10 minutes more.

Nutrition: Calories 150 Fat 9.7 g Carbohydrates 5.3 g Sugar 2.9 g Protein 11.2 g Cholesterol 255 mg

Spinach Tomato Frittata

Preparation Time:10 minutes

Cooking Time: 7 minutes

Servings:2

Ingredients:

- 2 eggs
- 1/4 cup fresh spinach, chopped
- 1/4 cup tomatoes, chopped
- 2 tbsp cream
- 1 tbsp cheddar cheese, grated

Directions:

1. Spray air fryer pan with cooking spray and set aside.
2. In a bowl, whisk eggs with remaining ingredients.
3. Pour egg mixture into the pan. Place pan in the air fryer basket and cook at 330 F for 7 minutes.

Nutrition: Calories 90 Fat 6.3 g Carbohydrates 1.8 g Sugar 1.2 g Protein 16.8 g Cholesterol 170 mg

Basil Feta Egg Bite

Preparation Time:10 minutes

Cooking Time: 5 minutes

Servings:7

Ingredients:

- 4 eggs
- 1 tbsp fresh basil, chopped
- 1/4 cup sun-dried tomatoes, diced
- 1/4 cup feta cheese, crumbled
- 1/2 cup cottage cheese, crumbled

Directions:

1. Spray egg mold with cooking spray and set aside.
2. In a bowl, beat eggs until frothy. Add remaining Ingredients into the eggs and stir to mix.
3. Pour egg mixture into the egg mold.
4. Place egg mold into the air fryer basket and cook at 330 F for 5 minutes.

Nutrition: Calories 66 Fat 4 g Carbohydrates 1.3 g Sugar 0.6 g Protein 6.2 g Cholesterol 100 mg

Cheese Garlicky Pork Chops

Preparation Time:10 minutes

Cooking Time: 20 minutes

Servings:8

Ingredients:

- 8 pork chops, boneless
- 3/4 cup parmesan cheese
- 2 tbsp butter, melted
- 2 tbsp coconut oil
- 1 tsp thyme
- 1 tbsp parsley
- 5 garlic cloves, minced
- 1/4 tsp pepper
- 1/2 tsp sea salt

Directions:

1. Spray air fryer basket with cooking spray.
2. Preheat the cosori air fryer to 400 F.
3. In a bowl, mix together butter, spices, parmesan cheese, and coconut oil.
4. Brush butter mixture on top of pork chops and place it into the air fryer basket and cook for 20 minutes. Turn pork chops halfway through.

5. Serve and enjoy.

Nutrition: Calories 344 Fat 28.2 g Carbohydrates 1.1 g Sugar 0 g Protein 21.2 g Cholesterol 83 mg

Garlic Lemon Pork Chops

Preparation Time:10 minutes

Cooking Time: 20 minutes

Servings:5

Ingredients:

- 2 lbs. pork chops
- 2 tbsp fresh lemon juice
- 2 tbsp garlic, minced
- 1 tbsp fresh parsley
- 1 1/2 tbsp olive oil
- Pepper
- Salt

Directions:

1. In a small bowl, mix together garlic, parsley, olive oil, and lemon juice. Season pork chops with pepper and salt.
2. Pour garlic mixture over the pork chops and coat well and allow to marinate for 30 minutes.
3. Add marinated pork chops into the air fryer basket and cook at 400 F for 20 minutes. Turn pork chops halfway through.
4. Serve and enjoy.

Nutrition: Calories 623 Fat 49.4 g Carbohydrates 1.3 g Sugar 0.2 g Protein 41.1 g Cholesterol 156 mg

Herb Cheese Pork Chops

Preparation Time:10 minutes

Cooking Time: 9 minutes

Servings:2

Ingredients:

- 2 pork chops, boneless
- 1 tsp paprika
- 3 tbsp parmesan cheese, grated
- 1/3 cup almond flour
- 1/2 tsp Cajun seasoning
- 1 tsp herb de Provence

Directions:

1. Preheat the cosori air fryer to 350 F.
2. Mix together almond flour, Cajun seasoning, herb de Provence, paprika, and parmesan cheese. Spray pork chops with cooking spray.
3. Coat pork chops with almond flour mixture and place into the air fryer basket and cook for 9 minutes.
4. Serve and enjoy.

Nutrition: Calories 360 Fat 27.3 g Carbohydrates 2.4 g Sugar 0.3 g Protein 26.7 g Cholesterol 85 mg

Creole Seasoned Pork Chops

Preparation Time:10 minutes

Cooking Time: 12 minutes

Servings:6

Ingredients:

- 1 1/2 lbs. pork chops, boneless
- 1 tsp garlic powder
- 1/4 cup parmesan cheese, grated
- 1/3 cup almond flour
- 1 tsp paprika
- 1 tsp Creole seasoning

Directions:

1. Spray air fryer basket with cooking spray.
2. Preheat the cosori air fryer to 360 F.
3. Add all ingredients except pork chops into the zip-lock bag.
4. Add pork chops into the bag. Seal bag and shake well.
5. Remove pork chops from the zip-lock bag and place it into the air fryer basket and cook for 12 minutes.
6. Serve and enjoy.

Nutrition: Calories 388 Fat 29.9 g Carbohydrates 1 g Sugar 0.2 g Protein 27.3 g Cholesterol 101 mg

Tender Pork Chops

Preparation Time:10 minutes

Cooking Time: 13 minutes

Servings:4

Ingredients:

- 4 pork chops, boneless
- 1/2 tsp granulated garlic
- 1/2 tsp celery seeds
- 1/2 tsp parsley
- 1/2 tsp granulated onion
- 2 tsp olive oil
- 1/2 tsp salt

Directions:

1. Spray air fryer basket with cooking spray.
2. In a small bowl, mix together with seasonings and sprinkle over the pork chops.
3. Place pork chops into the air fryer basket and cook at 350 F for 5 minutes. Turn pork chops and cook for 8 minutes more.
4. Serve and enjoy.

Nutrition: Calories 278 Fat 22.3 g Carbohydrates 0.4 g Sugar 0.1 g Protein 18.1 g Cholesterol 69 mg

Asian Pork Chops

Preparation Time:10 minutes

Cooking Time: 12 minutes

Servings:2

Ingredients:

- 2 pork chops
- 1 tsp black pepper
- 3 tbsp lemongrass, chopped
- 1 tbsp shallot, chopped
- 1 tbsp garlic, chopped
- 1 tsp liquid stevia
- 1 tbsp sesame oil
- 1 tbsp fish sauce
- 1 tsp soy sauce

Directions:

1. Add pork chops in a mixing bowl. Pour remaining Ingredients: over the pork chops and mix well. Place in refrigerator for 2 hours.
2. Preheat the cosori air fryer to 400 F.
3. Place marinated pork chops into the air fryer basket and cook for 12 minutes. Turn pork chops after 7 minutes.

4. Serve and enjoy.

Nutrition: Calories 340 Fat 26.8 g Carbohydrates 5.3 g Sugar 0.4 g Protein 19.3 g Cholesterol 69 mg

Easy & Delicious Pork Chops

Preparation Time:10 minutes

Cooking Time: 15 minutes

Servings:4

Ingredients:

- 4 pork chops
- 2 tsp parsley
- 2 tsp garlic, grated
- 1/4 tsp garlic powder
- 1/4 tsp onion powder
- 1 tbsp olive oil
- 1 tbsp butter
- Pepper
- Salt

Directions:

1. Preheat the cosori air fryer to 350 F.
2. In a large bowl, mix together seasonings, garlic, butter, and oil.
3. Add pork chops to the bowl and mix well. Place in refrigerator overnight.

4. Place marinated pork chops into the air fryer basket and cook for 15 minutes. Turn pork chops after 7 minutes.
5. Serve and enjoy.

Nutrition: Calories 315 Fat 26.3 g Carbohydrates 0.8 g Sugar 0.1 g Protein 18.2 g Cholesterol 76 mg

Dash Seasoned Pork Chops

Preparation Time:10 minutes

Cooking Time: 20 minutes

Servings:2

Ingredients:

- 2 pork chops, boneless
- 1 tbsp dash seasoning
- Pepper
- Salt

Directions:

1. Spray air fryer basket with cooking spray.
2. Rub seasoning all over the pork chops.
3. Place seasoned pork chops into the air fryer basket and cook at 360 F for 20 minutes. Turn halfway through.
4. Serve and enjoy.

Nutrition: Calories 256 Fat 19.9 g Carbohydrates 0 g Sugar 0 g Protein 18 g Cholesterol 69 mg

Easy Pork Butt

Preparation Time:10 minutes

Cooking Time: 20 minutes

Servings:4

Ingredients:

- 1 1/2 lbs. pork butt, chopped into pieces
- 1/4 cup jerk paste

Directions:

1. Spray air fryer basket with cooking spray.
2. Add meat and jerk paste into the bowl and coat well. Place in refrigerator overnight.
3. Preheat the cosori air fryer to 390 F.
4. Place marinated meat to the air fryer basket and cook for 20 minutes. Turn halfway through.
5. Serve and enjoy.

Nutrition: Calories 339 Fat 12.1 g Carbohydrates 0.8 g Sugar 0.6 g Protein 53 g Cholesterol 156 mg

Sweet and Sour Pork

Preparation Time: 25 minutes

Cooking Time: 12 minutes

Servings: 4

Ingredients:

- 2 pounds pork cut into chunks
- 2 large Eggs
- 1 tsp olive oil
- 1 cup cornstarch
- Salt and freshly ground black pepper to taste
- 1/4 tsp. Chinese spice
- Oil Mister

Directions:

1. Preheat the Power XL Air Fryer Grill by selecting grill mode
2. Adjust temperature to 350°F and Time to 5 minutes
3. Whisk egg and olive oil in a bowl
4. Add breadcrumbs to another bowl
5. Dip the beef schnitzel in the egg mixture.
6. then coat with the breadcrumb mixture
7. Arrange on the Power XL grilling plate

8. Transfer into the Power XL Air Fryer Grill

9. grill for 12 minutes, flipping halfway

10. Serve and enjoy!

11. Serving Suggestions: serve with ketchup or tomato sauce

12. Directions: & Cooking Tips: add spice to taste

Nutrition: Calories: 256kcal, Fat: 7g, Carb: 10g, Proteins: 21g

Pork Ratatouille

Preparation Time: 20 minutes

Cooking Time: 20 minutes

Servings: 4

Ingredients:

- 4 pork sausages
- For Ratatouille
- 1 pepper, chopped
- 15 oz tomatoes, chopped
- 2 zucchinis, chopped
- 1 red chili, chopped
- 1 eggplant, chopped
- 2 sprigs fresh thyme
- 1 medium red onion, chopped
- 1 tbsp. balsamic vinegar
- 2 garlic cloves, minced

Directions:

1. Preheat the Power XL Air Fryer Grill by selecting pizza/bake mode
2. Adjust temperature to 392°F and Time to 10 minutes
3. Combine zucchini, eggplant, onions, and oil in the cooking tray.

4. Transfer to the Power XL Air Fryer Grill, bake for 20 minutes
5. Remove and add the remaining Ratatouille ingredients.
6. Transfer to the Power XL Air Fryer Grill and cook for an additional 20 minutes
7. Remove and season with salt and pepper.
8. Add the sausage to the Pizza tray
9. Cook for 15 minutes, flipping halfway
10. Serve and enjoy
11. Serving Suggestions: Serve the sausage with the Ratatouille
12. Directions: & Cooking Tips: the vegetable must be well cooked

Nutrition: Calories: 233kcal, Fat: 11g, Carb: 4g, Proteins: 23g

Cheddar Pork Meatballs

The cheddar pork meatball is super delicious, succulent, and juicy. It is a creative way of putting your pork to good use.

Preparation Time: 25 minutes

Cooking Time: 10 minutes

Servings: 6

Ingredients:

- 1 lb. ground pork
- 1/2 tsp. maple syrup
- 1 large onion, chopped
- 2 tsp mustard
- Salt and black pepper to taste
- 1/2 cup chopped basil leaves
- 2 tbsp. grated cheddar cheese

Directions:

1. Preheat the Power XL Air Fryer Grill by selecting air fry mode
2. Adjust temperature to 390°F and Time to 5 minutes
3. Combine all the ingredients in a bowl.
4. Form into small balls
5. Arrange on the Air fryer baking tray

6. Transfer into the Power XL Air Fryer Grill

7. Air fry for 10 minutes, flip and cook for additional 5 minutes

8. Serve and enjoy!

9. Serving Suggestions: Serve with noodles and marinara sauce

10. Directions: & Cooking Tips: use an ice-cream scooper to form the balls

Nutrition: Calories: 300kcal, Fat: 24g, Carb: 3g, Proteins: 16g

Almond Pork Bite

Preparation Time: 25 minutes

Cooking Time: 20 minutes

Servings: 10

Ingredients:

- 16 oz. sausage meat
- 1 whole egg, beaten
- 1/3 cup chopped onion
- 2 tbsp. almonds, chopped
- 1/2 tsp pepper
- 2 tbsp. dried sage
- 1/3 cup sliced apples, sliced
- 1/2 tsp salt

Directions:

1. Preheat the Power XL Air Fryer Grill by selecting grill mode
2. Adjust temperature to 350°F and Time to 5 minutes
3. Combine all the ingredients in a bowl.
4. Pour into a Ziploc bag and marinate for 15 minutes
5. Form into cutlets

6. Arrange on the Power XL Air Fryer Grill grilling plate

7. Transfer into the Power XL Air Fryer Grill

8. Grill for 20 minutes

9. Serve and enjoy!

10. Serving Suggestions: Serve with heavy cream

11. Directions: & Cooking Tips: Drain the marinade

Nutrition: Calories: 391kcal, Fat: 16g, Carb: 32g, Proteins: 19g

Stuffed Pork Chops

Stuffed pork chops are the perfect recipe for a house party, can be ready in less than an hour, and the taste is just whoa!

Preparation Time: 30 minutes

Cooking Time: 20 minutes

Servings: 4

Ingredients:

- 8 pork chops
- 2 tbsp. olive
- 1/4 tsp. pepper
- 4 cups stuffing mix
- 1/2 tsp salt
- 4 garlic cloves, minced
- 2 tbsp sage leaves

Directions:

1. Preheat the Power XL Air Fryer Grill by selecting Air Fryer mode
2. Adjust temperature to 350°F and Time to 5 minutes
3. Cut a hole in the pork chops, fill the hole with stuffing mix

4. In a bowl, combine the remaining ingredients.
5. Add the pork chops and leave to marinate for 10 minutes
6. Arrange on the Power XL Air Fryer Grill grilling plate
7. Transfer into the Power XL Air Fryer Grill
8. Air fry for 20 minutes
9. Serve and enjoy!
10. Serving Suggestions: Serve with salad
11. Directions: & Cooking Tips: Drain the marinade

Nutrition: Calories: 300kcal, Fat: 13g, Carb: 19g, Proteins: 21g

Crispy Breaded Pork

Crispy breaded pork is tender meat that's has a crispy outside and a juicy inside

Preparation Time: 10 minutes

Cooking Time: 15 minutes

Servings: 6

Ingredients:

- 6 (3/4- inch thick) center-cut boneless pork chops
- olive oil spray
- 1-1/4 tsp. sweet paprika
- kosher salt
- 1/2 tsp onion powder
- 1 large egg, beaten
- 1/2 cup panko crumbs
- 1/3 cup crushed cornflakes crumbs
- 1/4 tsp. chili powder
- 2 tbsp. grated parmesan cheese
- 1/2 tsp garlic powder
- 1/8 tsp. black pepper

Directions:

1. Preheat the Power XL Air Fryer Grill by selecting Air Fryer mode

2. Adjust temperature to 390°F and Time to 5 minutes

3. Season the pork chops on both sides with salt

4. In a bowl, combine the remaining ingredients except for the egg.

5. Beat the egg in another bowl

6. Dip pork chops in eggs then in breadcrumb mixture

7. Arrange on the Air fryer baking tray, sprinkle with oil

8. Transfer into the Power XL Air Fryer Grill

9. Air fry for 6 minutes per sides

10. Serve and enjoy!

11. Serving Suggestions: serve with tomato sauce or ketchup

12. Directions: & Cooking Tips: you can dip the pork chops twice in the eggs and breadcrumb mixture

Nutrition: Calories: 281kcal, Fat: 12g, Carb: 7g, Proteins: 31g

Lemongrass Pork Chops

This lemongrass is known for the aroma and flavor they add to foods. This is not different as it gives the meal a nice fragrance

Preparation Time: 2 hours

Cooking Time: 10 minutes

Servings: 4

Ingredients:

- 3 pork chops
- 4 stalks lemongrass, trimmed and chopped
- 1-1/4 tsp. soy sauce
- 2 garlic cloves, minced
- 1-1/2 tbsp sugar
- 2 shallots, chopped
- 2 tbsp olive oil
- 1-1/4 tsp. fish sauce
- 1-1/2 tsp black pepper

Directions:

1. Combine all the ingredients in a bowl
2. add the pork chops and leave to marinate for 2 hours
3. Preheat the Power XL Air Fryer Grill by selecting Grill/air fry mode

4. Adjust temperature to 390°F and Time to 5 minutes

5. Remove the pork chops and arrange on the grilling plate

6. Transfer into the Power XL Air Fryer Grill

7. Air fry for 6 minutes, flip and air fry for additional 7 minutes

8. Serve and enjoy!

9. Serving Suggestions: serve with sautéed asparagus

10. Directions: & Cooking Tips: marinate for at least 2 hours to get a nice savory taste

Nutrition: Calories: 342kcal, Fat: 10g, Carb: 4g, Proteins: 30g

BBQ Pork Ribs

Preparing the BBQ pork Rib with the Power XL Air Fryer Grill produces a tender and juicy pork meat. The recipe can be for a small outdoor gathering

Preparation Time: 5 hours

Cooking Time: 25 minutes |

Servings: 3

Ingredients:

- 1 lb. pork ribs, cut into smaller pieces
- 1 tsp. soy sauce
- 1 tsp sesame oil
- 1 tsp oregano
- 1 tbsp Plus 1 tbsp maple syrup
- 3 tbsp barbecue sauce
- Salt and black pepper to taste
- 2 cloves garlic, minced
- 1 tbsp. cayenne pepper

Directions:

1. Combine all the ingredients in a bowl
2. add the pork chops and leave to marinate for 5 hours
3. Preheat the Power XL Air Fryer Grill by selecting Grill/ air fry mode

4. Adjust temperature to 390°F and Time to 5 minutes
5. Remove the pork chops and arrange on the grilling plate
6. Transfer into the Power XL Air Fryer Grill
7. Air fry for 15 minutes, flip and brush with the remaining 1 tbsp. maple syrup
8. air fry for additional 10 minutes
9. Serve and enjoy!
10. Serving Suggestions: Serve with maple syrup
11. Directions: & Cooking Tips: Drain the marinade

Nutrition: Calories: 346kcal, Fat: 11g, Carb: 5g, Proteins: 22g

Spicy Pork Chops

Preparation Time:10 minutes

Cooking Time: 10 minutes

Servings:4

Ingredients:

- 4 pork chops
- 1 1/2 tsp olive oil
- 1/2 tsp dried sage
- 1/4 tsp chili powder
- 1/2 tsp cayenne pepper
- 1/2 tsp black pepper
- 1/2 tsp ground cumin
- 1 tsp paprika
- 1/2 tsp garlic salt

Directions:

1. Preheat the cosori air fryer to 400 F.
2. In a small bowl, mix together paprika, garlic salt, sage, pepper, chili powder, cayenne pepper, and cumin.
3. Rub pork chops with spice mixture and place into the air fryer basket. Spray pork chops from the top with cooking spray.
4. Cook for 10 minutes. Turn halfway through.

Nutrition: Calories 277 Fat 21.9 g Carbohydrates 1.1 g Sugar 0.2 g Protein 18.3 g Cholesterol 69 mg

Easy Pork Patties

Preparation Time:10 minutes

Cooking Time: 35 minutes

Servings:6

Ingredients:

- 2 lbs. ground pork
- 1/2 cup almond flour
- 1 egg, lightly beaten
- 1 onion, minced
- 1 carrot, minced
- 1 tsp garlic powder
- 1 tsp paprika

Directions:

1. Add all Ingredients into the large bowl and mix until well combined.
2. Make small patties from meat mixture and place into the air fryer basket and cook at 375 F for 20 minutes.
3. Turn pork patties and cook for 15 minutes more.

Nutrition: Calories 254 Fat 7.3 g Carbohydrates 3.8 g Sugar 1.6 g Protein 41.4 g Cholesterol 138 mg

Lemon Pepper Seasoned Pork Chops

Preparation Time:10 minutes

Cooking Time: 15 minutes

Servings:4

Ingredients:

- 4 pork chops, boneless
- 1 tsp lemon pepper seasoning
- Salt

Directions:

1. Season pork chops with lemon pepper seasoning, and salt.
2. Place pork chops into the air fryer basket and cook at 400 F for 15 minutes.

Nutrition: Calories 257 Fat 19.9 g Carbohydrates 0.3 g Sugar 0 g Protein 18 g Cholesterol 69 mg

Flavorful Pork Chops

Preparation Time:10 minutes

Cooking Time: 16 minutes

Servings:4

Ingredients:

- 4 pork chops, boneless
- 2 tsp olive oil
- 1/2 tsp celery seed
- 1/2 tsp parsley
- 1/2 tsp onion powder
- 1/2 tsp garlic powder
- 1/2 tsp salt

Directions:

1. Brush pork chops with olive oil.
2. Mix together celery seed, parsley, onion powder, garlic powder, and salt and sprinkle over pork chops.
3. Place pork chops into the air fryer basket and cook at 350 F for 16 minutes. Turn pork chops halfway through.

Nutrition: Calories 279 Fat 22.3 g Carbohydrates 0.6 g Sugar 0.2 g Protein 18.1 g Cholesterol 69 mg

BBQ Pork Chops

Preparation Time:10 minutes

Cooking Time: 14 minutes

Servings:2

Ingredients:

- 2 pork chops
- 1/2 tsp sesame oil
- 1/4 cup BBQ sauce, sugar-free
- 2 garlic cloves, minced

Directions:

1. Spray air fryer basket with cooking spray.
2. Preheat the cosori air fryer to 350 F.
3. Add all Ingredients into the mixing bowl and mix well and place in the fridge for 1 hour.
4. Place marinated pork chops into the air fryer basket and cook for 14 minutes. Turn halfway through.
5. Serve and enjoy.

Nutrition: Calories 317 Fat 21.1 g Carbohydrates 12.4 g Sugar 8.2 g Protein 18.2 g Cholesterol 69 mg

Pesto Pork Chops

Preparation Time:10 minutes

Cooking Time: 18 minutes

Servings:5

Ingredients:

- 5 pork chops
- 1 tbsp basil pesto
- 2 tbsp almond flour
- Pepper
- Salt

Directions:

1. Spray pork chops with cooking spray.
2. Rub basil pesto on top of pork chops and coat with almond flour.
3. Place pork chops into the air fryer basket and cook at 350 F for 18 minutes.
4. Serve and enjoy.

Nutrition: Calories 320 Fat 25.5 g Carbohydrates 2.4 g Sugar 0.4 g Protein 20.4 g Cholesterol 69 mg

Coconut Butter Pork Chops

Preparation Time:10 minutes

Cooking Time: 15 minutes

Servings:2

Ingredients:

- 4 pork chops
- 1 tbsp coconut oil
- 1 tbsp coconut butter
- 2 tsp parsley
- 2 tsp garlic, grated
- Pepper
- Salt

Directions:

1. Preheat the cosori air fryer to 350 F.
2. In a large bowl, mix together garlic, butter, coconut oil, parsley, pepper, and salt.
3. Rub garlic mixture over the pork chops. Wrap marinated pork chops into the foil and place it in the refrigerator for 1 hour.
4. Remove pork chops from foil and place into the air fryer basket and cook for 15 minutes. Turn pork chops after 7 minutes.
5. Serve and enjoy.

Nutrition: Calories 686 Fat 57.1 g Carbohydrates 5 g Sugar 1 g Protein 37.2 g Cholesterol 138 mg

Crispy Pork Chops

Preparation Time:10 minutes

Cooking Time: 20 minutes

Servings:4

Ingredients:

- 4 pork chops, boneless
- 2 eggs, lightly beaten
- 1 cup almond flour
- 1/4 cup parmesan cheese, grated
- 1 tbsp onion powder
- 1 tbsp garlic powder
- 1/2 tbsp black pepper
- 1/2 tsp sea salt

Directions:

1. Spray air fryer basket with cooking spray.
2. Preheat the cosori air fryer to 350 F.
3. In a shallow bowl, mix together almond flour, parmesan cheese, onion powder, garlic powder, pepper, and salt.
4. Whisk eggs in a shallow dish.
5. Dip pork chops into the egg then coat with almond flour mixture.

6. Place coated pork chops into the air fryer basket and cook for 20 minutes. Turn pork chops halfway through.
7. Serve and enjoy.

Nutrition: Calories 363 Fat 27 g Carbohydrates 5.3 g Sugar 1.6 g Protein 24.9 g Cholesterol 155 mg

Air Fryer Beef Steak

Preparation Time: 10 minutes

Cooking Time: 10 minutes |

Servings: 4

Ingredients:

- 2 lb. Ribeye steak
- Salt and pepper to taste
- 1 tbsp. Olive oil

Directions:

1. Preheat the Power XL Air Fryer Grill by selecting air fry mode
2. Adjust temperature to 356°F and Timer to 5 minutes
3. Season the steak with olive oil, salt, and pepper.
4. Place on the Air fryer pizza tray
5. Transfer into the Power XL Air Fryer Grill
6. Air fry for 7 minutes, flip and cook for additional 6 minutes
7. Serve and enjoy
8. Serving Suggestions: Serve with any sauce of choice

9. Directions: & Cooking Tips: leave the steak to marinate for some minutes

Nutrition: Calories: 230kcal, Fat: 17g, Carb: 1g, Proteins: 23g

Air Fryer Meatballs

Preparation Time: 10 minutes

Cooking Time: 20 minutes |

Servings: 4

Ingredients:

- 2 lb. Ground beef
- 2cloves garlic, minced
- 2 tbsp. Chopped parsley
- 2 eggs
- Salt and black pepper to taste
- 1-1/2 cup grated parmesan cheese
- 1/4 cup of minced onions
- 1/2 tsp. red pepper flakes
- 1/2 tsp. Italian seasoning

Directions:

1. Preheat the Power XL Air Fryer Grill by selecting air fry mode
2. Adjust temperature to 350°F and Time to 5 minutes
3. Combine all the ingredients in a bowl.
4. Form into small balls
5. Arrange on the Air fryer baking tray
6. Transfer into the Power XL Air Fryer Grill

7. Air fry for 8 minutes, flip and cook for additional 5 minutes

8. Serve and enjoy!

9. Serving Suggestions: Serve with sauce or dips

10. Directions: & Cooking Tips: make sure the ingredients are well combined

Nutrition: Calories: 321kcal, Fat: 15g, Carb: 3g, Proteins: 35g

Mushroom Meatloaf

Preparation Time: 20 minutes

Cooking Time: 10 minutes |

Servings: 4

Ingredients:

- 14 oz. Lean ground beef
- 1 chorizo sausage, chopped
- 1 egg
- 1 small onion, chopped
- Salt and freshly ground black pepper, to taste
- 3 Tbsp. Olive oil
- 2 tbsp. fresh mushrooms, sliced thinly
- 1 garlic clove, minced
- 2 tbsp. fresh cilantro, chopped
- 3 tbsp breadcrumbs

Directions:

- Preheat the Power XL Air Fryer Grill by selecting pizza/bake mode
- Adjust temperature to 390°F and Time to 10 minutes
- Combine all the ingredients in a bowl except the mushroom.

- Pour into the Air fryer baking tray, smoothen with a spatula
- Arrange the mushroom on top
- Transfer into the Power XL Air Fryer Grill
- Bake for 25 minutes
- Serve and enjoy!
- Serving Suggestions: garnish with cilantro
- Directions: & Cooking Tips: make sure all the ingredients are well combined

Nutrition: Calories: 200kcal, Fat: 6g, Carb: 26g, Proteins: 18g

Cheese Stuffed Meatballs

Preparation Time: 10 minutes

Cooking Time: 10 minutes

Servings: 2

Ingredients:

- 1/3 cup bread crumbs
- 1 lb. Lean ground beef
- 1 egg
- 3 tbsps. milk
- 1/2 tsp. Marjoram
- 1 tbsp ketchup
- salt and freshly ground black pepper
- 20 (1/2-inch) cubes of cheese
- Olive oil for misting

Directions:

1. Preheat the Power XL Air Fryer Grill by selecting air fry mode
2. Adjust temperature to 390°F and Time to 10 minutes
3. Combine all the ingredients in a bowl except cheese.
4. Form 20 meatballs.
5. Shape each meatball around the cheese

6. Arrange in the Air fryer baking tray.

7. Transfer into the Power XL Air Fryer Grill

8. Bake for 15 minutes

9. Serve and enjoy

10. Serving Suggestions: sprinkle with cheese

11. Directions: & Cooking Tips: serve with marinara sauce

Nutrition: Calories: 321kcal, Fat: 12g, Carb: 16g, Proteins: 19g

Carrot and Beef Cocktail Balls

Preparation Time: 40 minutes

Cooking Time: 10 minutes |

Servings: 4

Ingredients:

- 1 lb. ground beef
- 2 carrots,
- 1 red onion, peeled and chopped
- 3/4 cup breadcrumbs
- Salt and black pepper to taste
- 1/2 tsp dried rosemary, crushed
- 2 cloves garlic, minced
- 1/2 tsp dried basil
- 1 Egg
- 1 tsp dried oregano

Directions:

1. Pulse carrot, onion, and garlic in a food processor
2. Pour into a bowl, add the remaining ingredients except for flour
3. Form into a ball, refrigerate for 20 minutes

4. Roll in flour and arrange on the Air fryer baking tray

5. Transfer to the Power XL Air Fryer Grill and select the air fryer mode.

6. Adjust temperature to 390°F

7. Set Time to 20 minutes

8. Serve with toothpicks

9. Serving Suggestions: serve with sauce, garnish with parsley

10. Directions: & Cooking Tips: pulse the carrot until smooth

Nutrition: Calories: 224kcal, Fat: 6g, Carb: 29g, Proteins: 10g

Marinated Cajun Beef

Preparation Time: 60 minutes

Cooking Time: 25 minutes|

Servings: 2

Ingredients:

- 1lb. Beef tenderloins
- 1/3 cup beef broth
- 1/2 tsp. garlic powder
- 2 tbsp Cajun seasoning, crushed
- 1-1/2 tbsp. Olive oil
- 1/2 tbsp pear cider vinegar
- 1/3 tsp cayenne pepper
- 1 tsp. Salt
- 1 tsp. Freshly ground black pepper

Directions:

1. Add all the Ingredients: to a bowl.
2. Add the beef and leave to marinate for 40 minutes
3. Place on the Air fryer pizza tray
4. Transfer to the Power XL Air Fryer Grill
5. Select the air fryer/grill mode
6. Adjust temperature to 390°F

7. Grill for 22 minutes, flipping halfway through
8. Serve and enjoy
9. Serving Suggestions: serve with tomato sauce
10. Directions: & Cooking Tips: Drain the marinade

Nutrition: Calories: 287kcal, Fat: 23g, Carb: 8g, Proteins: 48g

Beef and Potatoes

Preparation Time: 10 minutes

Cooking Time: 15 minutes

Servings: 2

Ingredients:

- 1 lb. Ground beef
- 3 cups of mashed potatoes
- 1 cup sour cream
- 2 eggs
- 2 tbsp. Garlic powder

Directions:

1. Preheat the Power XL Air Fryer Grill by selecting bake/pizza mode
2. Adjust temperature to 350°F and Time to 5 minutes
3. Combine all the ingredients in a bowl.
4. Pour into the Air fryer baking tray
5. Transfer into the Power XL Air Fryer Grill
6. Bake for 6 minutes
7. Serve and enjoy!
8. Serving Suggestions: serve any toppings of choice

9. Directions: & Cooking Tips: combine all the Ingredients:

Nutrition: Calories: 320kcal, Fat: 7g, Carb: 9g, Proteins: 27g

Breaded Beef Schnitzel

Preparation Time: 10 minutes

Cooking Time: 10 minutes|

Servings: 2

Ingredients:

- 4 beef schnitzel
- 2 tbsp. Olive oil
- 1 egg
- 5 cups of breadcrumbs

Directions:

1. Preheat the Power XL Air Fryer Grill by selecting grill mode
2. Adjust temperature to 350°F and Time to 5 minutes
3. Whisk egg and olive oil in a bowl
4. Add breadcrumbs to another bowl
5. Dip the beef schnitzel in the egg mixture.
6. then coat with the breadcrumb mixture
7. Arrange on the grilling plate
8. Transfer into the Power XL Air Fryer Grill
9. Grill for 12 minutes, flipping halfway
10. Serve and enjoy!
11. Serving Suggestions: serve with ketchup

12. Directions: & Cooking Tips: drain the
      beef schnitzel

Nutrition: Calories: 256kcal, Fat: 5g, Carb: 12g,
Proteins: 15g

Quick & Easy Steak Tips

Preparation Time:10 minutes

Cooking Time: 6 minutes

Servings:3

Ingredients:

- 1 1/2 lbs. steak, cut into 3/4-inch cubes
- 1/8 tsp cayenne
- 1 tsp Montreal steak seasoning
- 1/2 tsp garlic powder
- 1 tsp olive oil

Directions:

1. Spray air fryer basket with cooking spray.
2. Preheat the cosori air fryer to 400 F.
3. Toss steak cubes with oil, cayenne, steak seasoning, garlic powder, pepper, and salt.
4. Add steak cubes into the air fryer basket and cook for 4-6 minutes.

Nutrition: Calories 469 Fat 12.9 g Carbohydrates 0.4 g Sugar 0.1 g Protein 82 g Cholesterol 204 mg

Simple Sirloin Steaks

Preparation Time: 10 minutes

Cooking Time: 12 minutes

Servings: 2

Ingredients:

- 2 sirloin steaks
- 2 tbsp steak seasoning
- Directions:
- Spray steaks with cooking spray and season with steak seasoning.
- Place steaks into the air fryer basket and cook at 400 F for 12 minutes. Turn steaks halfway through.

Nutrition: Calories 334 Fat 11.2 g Carbohydrates 0 g Sugar 0 g Protein 54.6 g Cholesterol 161 mg

Flavorful Steak

Preparation Time:10 minutes

Cooking Time: 18 minutes

Servings:2

Ingredients:

- 2 steaks, rinsed and pat dry with a paper towel
- 1 tsp olive oil
- 1/2 tsp garlic powder
- 1/4 tsp onion powder

Directions:

1. Rub steaks with oil and season with garlic powder, onion powder, pepper, and salt.
2. Place steaks into the air fryer basket and cook at 400 F for 18 minutes. Turn steaks halfway through.

Nutrition: Calories 252 Fat 8.1 g Carbohydrates 0.8 g Sugar 0.3 g Protein 41.7 g Cholesterol 104 mg

Italian Beef Roast

Preparation Time:10 minutes

Cooking Time: 45 minutes

Servings:6

Ingredients:

- 2 1/2 lbs. beef roast
- 2 tbsp Italian seasoning
- 1 tsp olive oil

Directions:

1. Rub beef roast with oil and season with Italian seasoning, pepper, and salt.
2. Place the beef roast into the air fryer basket and cook at 350 F for 45 minutes.
3. Slice and serve.

Nutrition: Calories 372 Fat 13.9 g Carbohydrates 0.5 g Sugar 0.4 g Protein 57.4 g Cholesterol 172 mg

Rosemary Thyme Beef Roast

Preparation Time:10 minutes

Cooking Time: 15 minutes

Servings:4

Ingredients:

- 2 lbs. beef roast
- 1 tsp dried rosemary
- 1 tsp dried thyme
- 1/4 tsp onion powder
- 1 tsp olive oil

Directions:

1. Rub beef roast with oil and season with rosemary, thyme, onion powder, pepper, and salt.
2. Place the beef roast into the air fryer basket and cook at 390 F for 15 minutes. Turn roast after 10 minutes.
3. Slice and serve.

Nutrition: Calories 434 Fat 15.4 g Carbohydrates 0.5 g Sugar 0.1 g Protein 68.9 g Cholesterol 203 mg

Italian Meatballs

Preparation Time:10 minutes

Cooking Time: 11 minutes

Servings:4

Ingredients:

- 1 egg
- 1 lb. ground beef
- 1 tsp Italian seasoning
- 1 tbsp onion, minced
- 1/4 cup marinara sauce, sugar-free
- 1/3 cup parmesan cheese, shredded
- 1 tsp garlic, minced

Directions:

1. Spray air fryer basket with cooking spray.
2. Add all Ingredients into the mixing bowl and mix until well combined.
3. Make meatballs from mixture and place into the air fryer basket and cook at 350 F for 12 minutes.

Nutrition: Calories 274 Fat 10.8 g Carbohydrates 3.2 g Sugar 1.7 g Protein 38.9 g Cholesterol 150 mg

Burgers Patties

Preparation Time:10 minutes

Cooking Time: 10 minutes

Servings:2

Ingredients:

- 1/2 lb. ground beef
- 1/4 tsp onion powder
- 1/4 tsp garlic powder
- 2 drops liquid smoke
- 1/2 tsp hot sauce
- 1/2 tsp dried parsley
- 1/4 tsp black pepper
- 1/2 tbsp Worcestershire sauce
- 1/4 tsp salt

Directions:

1. Spray air fryer basket with cooking spray.
2. Add all Ingredients into the large mixing bowl and mix until combined.
3. Make patties from mixture and place into the air fryer basket and cook at 350 F for 10 minutes. Turn patties halfway through.

Nutrition: Calories 218 Fat 7.1 g Carbohydrates 1.5 g Sugar 1 g Protein 34.5 g Cholesterol 101 mg

Tasty Beef Patties

Preparation Time:10 minutes

Cooking Time: 10 minutes

Servings:2

Ingredients:

- 1/2 lb. ground beef
- 1 tsp ginger, minced
- 1/2 tbsp soy sauce
- 1 tbsp gochujang
- 1/4 tsp salt
- 1 tbsp green onion, chopped
- 1/2 tbsp sesame oil

Directions:

1. In a large bowl, mix together ground beef and remaining ingredients. Place mixture in the refrigerator for 1 hour.
2. Make patties from beef mixture and place into the air fryer basket and cook at 360 F for 10 minutes.

Nutrition: Calories 257 Fat 10.5 g Carbohydrates 3.3 g Sugar 1.5 g Protein 35 g Cholesterol 101 mg

Meatloaf

Preparation Time: 10 minutes

Cooking Time: 15 minutes

Servings: 2

Ingredients:

- 1 egg
- 1/2 lb. ground beef
- 1/2 tsp turmeric
- 1 tsp garam masala
- 1/2 tbsp garlic, minced
- 1/2 tbsp ginger, minced
- 1 tbsp cilantro, chopped
- 1/8 tsp ground cardamom
- 1/4 tsp ground cinnamon
- 1/2 tsp cayenne
- 1/2 cup onion, chopped
- 1/2 tsp salt

Directions:

1. In a large bowl, mix together all the ingredients until well combined.
2. Place meat mixture into air fryer safe pan and place in the air fryer basket.
3. Cook at 360 F for 15 minutes.

4. Slice and serve.

Nutrition: Calories 266 Fat 9.5 g Carbohydrates 5.5 g Sugar 1.5 g Protein 37.9 g Cholesterol 183 mg

Tender & Juicy Kebab

Preparation Time:10 minutes

Cooking Time: 10 minutes

Servings:2

Ingredients:

- 1/2 lb. ground beef
- 1 tbsp parsley, chopped
- 1/2 tbsp olive oil
- 1 tbsp kabab spice mix
- 1/2 tbsp garlic, minced
- 1/2 tsp salt

Directions:

1. Add all Ingredients into the stand mixer until well combined.
2. Equally, divide the meat mixture into two portions and make two sausage shapes.
3. Place kababs into the air fryer basket and cook at 370 F for 10 minutes.

Nutrition: Calories 259 Fat 11.1 g Carbohydrates 2.7 g Sugar 1.1 g Protein 35.2 g Cholesterol 101 mg

Meatloaf De Luxe

Preparation Time:10 minutes

Cooking Time: 25 minutes

Servings:2

Ingredients:

- 1/2 lb. ground beef
- 1 tbsp chorizo, chopped
- 1 1/2 tbsp breadcrumbs
- 1 egg, lightly beaten
- 1 mushroom, sliced
- 1/2 tbsp fresh thyme
- 1/2 small onion, chopped

Directions:

1. Preheat the cosori air fryer at 400 F.
2. In a large bowl, mix together all ingredients until well combined.
3. Transfer meat mixture into the air fryer safe pan.
4. Place pan into the air fryer basket and cook for 25 minutes.
5. Slice and serve.

Nutrition: Calories 337 Fat 15.1 g Carbohydrates 6.5 g Sugar 1.4 g Protein 41.8 g Cholesterol 196 mg

Meatballs Surprise

Preparation Time:10 minutes

Cooking Time: 20 minutes

Servings:2

Ingredients:

- 1/2 lb. ground beef
- 2 tbsp onion, chopped
- 1 1/2 tbsp mushrooms, diced
- 1 tbsp parsley, chopped
- 1/4 cup almond flour
- 1/4 tsp pepper
- 1/2 tsp salt

Directions:

1. In a mixing bowl, combine together all ingredients until well combined.
2. Make meatballs from mixture and place into the air fryer basket and cook at 350 F for 20 minutes.

Nutrition: Calories 237 Fat 8.9 g Carbohydrates 2.1 g Sugar 0.6 g Protein 35.5 g Cholesterol 101 mg

Marinated Steak

Preparation Time:10 minutes

Cooking Time: 7 minutes

Servings:2

Ingredients:

- 12 oz steaks
- 1 tbsp Montreal steak seasoning
- 1 tsp liquid smoke
- 1 tbsp soy sauce
- 1/2 tbsp cocoa powder

Directions :

1. Add steak and remaining Ingredients into the large zip-lock bag. Shake well and place it in the refrigerator overnight.
2. Spray air fryer basket with cooking spray.
3. Place marinated steaks into the air fryer basket and cook at 375 F for 5 minutes.
4. Turn steak and cook for 2 minutes more.

Nutrition: Calories 356 Fat 8.7 g Carbohydrates 1.4 g Sugar 0.2 g Protein 62.2 g Cholesterol 153 mg

Asian Beef

Preparation Time:10 minutes

Cooking Time: 20 minutes

Servings:4

Ingredients:

- 1 lb. flank steak, sliced
- 1 tsp xanthan gum
- For sauce:
- 1 tsp ground ginger
- 1 tbsp chili sauce
- 1 garlic clove, crushed
- 2 tbsp white wine vinegar
- 1 tbsp water
- 1 tbsp arrowroot powder
- 1/2 tsp sesame seeds
- 1 tsp liquid stevia
- 1/2 cup soy sauce

Directions:

1. Toss sliced meat with xanthan gum.
2. Spray air fryer basket with cooking spray.
3. Add meat into the air fryer basket and cook at 390 F for 20 minutes. Turn meat halfway through.

4. Meanwhile, add remaining Ingredients into the saucepan and heat over low heat until begins to boil.
5. Add cooked meat to the sauce and coat well.
6. Serve and enjoy.

Nutrition: Calories 253 Fat 9.7 g Carbohydrates 6.2 g Sugar 0.7 g Protein 33.8 g Cholesterol 62 mg

Flavorful Beef Roast

Preparation Time:10 minutes

Cooking Time: 45 minutes

Servings:8

Ingredients:

- 2 1/2 lbs. beef roast
- 1/2 tsp onion powder
- 1 tsp rosemary
- 1 tsp dill
- 2 tbsp olive oil
- 1/2 tsp black pepper
- 1/2 tsp garlic powder

Directions:

1. Preheat the cosori air fryer to 360 F.
2. Mix together black pepper, garlic powder, onion powder, rosemary, dill, and olive oil. Rub all over the beef roast.
3. Place beef roast in the air fryer basket and cook for 45 minutes.
4. Serve and enjoy.

Nutrition: Calories 296 Fat 12.4 g Carbohydrates 0.5 g Sugar 0.1 g Protein 43.1 g Cholesterol 127 mg

Cheese Butter Steak

Preparation Time:10 minutes

Cooking Time: 8 minutes

Servings:2

Ingredients:

- 2 ribeye steaks
- 2 tbsp blue cheese butter
- 1 tsp black pepper
- 2 tsp garlic powder
- 2 tsp kosher salt

Directions:

1. Preheat the cosori air fryer to 400 F.
2. Spray air fryer basket with cooking spray.
3. Mix together garlic powder, pepper, and salt and rub all over the steaks.
4. Place steak in the air fryer basket and cook for 8 minutes. Turn steak halfway through.
5. Top with blue butter cheese and serve.

Nutrition: Calories 222 Fat 15 g Carbohydrates 4.1 g Sugar 0.7 g Protein 18 g Cholesterol 6 mg

Tasty Ginger Garlic Beef

Preparation Time:10 minutes

Cooking Time: 20 minutes

Servings:4

Ingredients:

- 1 lb. beef tips, sliced
- 1 tbsp ginger, sliced
- 2 tbsp garlic, minced
- 2 tbsp sesame oil
- 1 tbsp fish sauce
- 2 tbsp coconut aminos
- 1 tsp xanthan gum
- 1/4 cup scallion, chopped
- 2 red chili peppers, sliced
- 2 tbsp water

Directions:

1. Spray air fryer basket with cooking spray.
2. Toss beef with xanthan gum together.
3. Add beef into the air fryer basket and cook at 390F for 20 minutes. Turn halfway through.
4. Meanwhile, in a saucepan add remaining ingredients except for green onion and heat

over low heat. Once it begins boiling then remove from heat.

5. Add cooked meat into the saucepan and stir to coat. Let sit in the saucepan for 5 minutes.

6. Transfer in serving dish and top with green onion and serve.

Nutrition: Calories 349 Fat 21.9 g Carbohydrates 5.7 g Sugar 0.5 g Protein 31.4 g Cholesterol 93 mg

Beef Strip with Snow Pea and Mushrooms

Preparation Time:8 Minutes

Cooking Time: 22 Minutes

Servings: 2

Ingredients:

- 2 beef steaks (cut into strips)
- 2 tbsp. soy sauce
- 7 oz. snow pea
- 1 medium yellow onion (cut into rings)
- 1 tbsp. olive oil
- 8 oz. white mushroom (cut into halves)
- Salt and black pepper to taste

Directions:

1. Preheat the air fryer to 3500F.
2. Pour the olive oil and soy sauce, into a bowl then whisk. Toss in the beef strip to coat.
3. In a separate bowl, mix the mushroom, snow pea, onions, salt, and pepper. Transfer the contents in the bowl to a pan and fit it into the air fryer. Set the Timer for 16 minutes and start cooking.

4. Turn up the air fryer's temperature to 4000F, add the beef strip, and cook for another 6 minutes.

5. Serve.

Nutrition: Calories: 231kcal, Fat: 7g, Carb: 14 g, Proteins: 23g

Beef Fillet with Garlic Mayo

Preparation Time:10 Minutes

Cooking Time: 40 Minutes

Servings: 8

Ingredients:

- 3 lb. beef fillet
- 1 cup mayonnaise
- 4 tbsp. Dijon mustard
- 1/3 cup sour cream
- 1/4 cup chopped tarragon
- 2 tbsp. chopped chives
- 2 cloves garlic (minced)
- Salt and black pepper, to taste

Directions:

1. Preheat the air fryer to 3700F.
2. Season beef using salt and pepper, transfer to the air fryer, and cook for 20 minutes. Remove and set aside.
3. In a bowl, whisk the mustard and tarragon. Add the beef and toss, return to the air fryer and cook for 20 minutes.

4. In a separate bowl, mix the garlic, sour cream, mayonnaise, chives, salt, and pepper. Whisk and set aside.

5. Serve the beef with the garlic-mayo spread.

Nutrition: Calories: 400kcal, Fat: 12g, Carb: 26g, Proteins: 19g

www.ingramcontent.com/pod-product-compliance
Lightning Source LLC
Chambersburg PA
CBHW050219270326
41914CB00003BA/482